Radiant Skin

Radiant Skin

By Health Is Luxury

ISBN: 979-8-9922102-3-1

For permission requests, please contact Health Is Luxury at:
Email: yourHealthIsLuxury@gmail.com
Website: www.HealthIsLuxury.org

Published by Health Is Luxury.
This book is intended to educate and inform readers about skincare and related topics.

Disclaimer

The information contained in this book is for educational and informational purposes only and is not intended as medical advice. The content reflects the author's research, opinions, and experience. Readers should consult with a qualified healthcare professional regarding any medical conditions or concerns related to skincare.

Health Is Luxury and the author are not responsible for any adverse effects, misuse, or outcomes arising from the use of the information or products mentioned in this book. The mention of any specific product or ingredient does not constitute endorsement or recommendation unless explicitly stated.

All product formulations and recipes mentioned in this book are intended for informational purposes and should be tested appropriately before use. Readers are encouraged to conduct their own research and use their discretion when selecting skincare products.

Table of Contents

Introduction: The Joy of Radiant Skin

- Understanding Skin Types
- Choosing the Right Soaps

Chapter 1: Understanding Your Skin

- The Structure of Skin: Layers and Functions
- The Skin's Natural Barrier
- Common Skin Types and Their Needs

Chapter 2: Factors Contributing to Healthy Skin

- Skin and Skin Nutrition
- The Role of Vitamins and Minerals
- Hydration: Inside and Out

Chapter 3: The Importance of Blood Health in Skin Care

- Blood's Role in Nourishing Skin
- What Contributes to Healthy Blood
- How Toxins and Poor Diet Affect Blood and Skin Health
- How Clean Blood Leads to Clear, Radiant Skin
- Practical Tips for Keeping Your Blood Clean
- Skin Conditions Linked to Poor Blood Health
- Natural Methods to Cleanse the Blood
- The Role of Antioxidants in Blood Health

Chapter 4: Maintaining Skin Health Naturally

- The Skin's Natural Barrier and Why It Matters
- The Dangers of EDTA and Synthetic Chemicals
- Other Harmful Toxins Found in Commercial Skin Care Products
- The Benefits of Natural Soaps
- How Toxins in Public Water Impact Your Skin
- How Natural Ingredients Combat Environmental Toxins

Chapter 5: Herbs, Vitamins, and Natural Ingredients for Radiant Skin

- Vitamins for Healthy, Glowing Skin
- Herbs for Radiant Skin
- Natural Oils and Butters for Skin Health

Chapter 6: The Role of All-Natural Soaps in Skin Care

- Why Synthetic Soaps Harm the Skin
- Health Is Luxury: Crafting the World's Best Soaps
- How to Make Your Skin Beautiful, Soft, and Radiant

Chapter 7: External and Environmental Factors Affecting Skin Health

- Excessive Sun Exposure and Skin Damage
- Pollution and Toxins
- Invisible Skin Aggressors
- The Gift of Melanin
- The Pineal Gland: Powerhouse of Melanin Production
- Nutritional Support for Melanin Production
- Vitamins and Supplements for Melanin-Rich Skin
- Toxic Skin Care Ingredients That Damage Melanin Production
- Protecting and Nourishing Melanin-Rich Skin Naturally
- The Power of Melanin

Chapter 8: Internal Factors: Gut Health and Skin Health

- The Gut-Skin Axis: How They Communicate
- Foods That Promote Glowing Skin
- Detoxification for Clear Skin
- The Importance of Gut-Brain-Skin Communication

Chapter 9: Blood Cleansing for Optimum Skin Health

- The Importance of Blood Cleansing for Skin Health
- Chlorophyll-Rich Foods for Blood Purification
- Green Drinks for Skin Health
- Intermittent Fasting for Blood Cleansing and Skin Health
- Antioxidants for Healthy Blood and Skin
- Additional Natural Practices to Cleanse the Blood

Chapter 10: Anti-Aging Through Natural Skin Care

- Natural Antioxidants for Youthful Skin
- Reversing Damage Naturally
- Building a Routine for Youthful Skin
- The Power of Meditation for Youthful Skin
- How Stress Affects Skin
- Meditation for Anti-Aging

Chapter 11: The Holistic Approach to Skin Care

- The Mind-Body-Skin Connection
- How to Manage Stress for Healthy Skin
- The Power of Sleep
- Tips for Optimizing Sleep for Better Skin
- Holistic Skin Care
- Mindfulness in Skin Care

Introduction: The Joy of Radiant Skin

Welcome to **Radiant Skin** by **Health Is Luxury,** where we believe that beautiful, healthy skin is one of life's simple joys. Your skin is much more than just the surface others see—it's your body's first line of defense, a reflection of your internal well-being, and a source of confidence when it's nourished and glowing. Taking care of your skin should feel like a daily ritual of self-care, bringing moments of empowerment and happiness to your routine.

We know that maintaining radiant, healthy skin can be easy, fun, and rewarding—especially when you use products made from nature's finest ingredients. That's why we're here to guide you on a journey of skin care that's as luxurious as it is pure, using herbs, vitamins, and our handcrafted, all-natural soaps that cleanse, nourish, and protect.

Each chapter of this book is designed to offer you simple yet powerful insights into how you can care for your skin naturally, from understanding your skin type to choosing the right soap, and from exploring the role of natural ingredients to finding joy in every step of your skincare routine.

Understanding Skin Types and Choosing the Right Soap

At **Health Is Luxury**, we believe that every skin type deserves the purest, most natural care. Whether your skin is dry, oily, sensitive, or a combination, our handcrafted soaps are designed to meet your skin's unique needs. Let's explore the different skin types and recommend which of our luxurious soaps is best suited for you.

Normal Skin

If you're one of the lucky ones with **normal skin**, your complexion is naturally well-balanced—not too oily or too dry, and with few imperfections. Your skin's harmony deserves to be maintained with gentle care, using products that support its natural radiance without disrupting its delicate balance.

- **Recommended Soap: 50:50 Butter**
  - **Why It Works**: Our **50:50 Butter** soap is the simplest and purest formulation, containing only two ingredients—**organic shea butter** and **coconut oil**. This soap provides gentle cleansing while keeping your skin soft, smooth, and perfectly hydrated. It's the ideal choice for maintaining normal skin's natural glow, day after day.

Dry Skin

For those with **dry skin**, your skin might often feel tight, rough, or flaky, craving deep hydration. You deserve a soap that replenishes moisture and helps restore your skin's softness, leaving it feeling nourished and cared for.

- **Recommended Soap: Rose Butter**
    - **Why It Works**: The **Rose Butter** soap is a luxurious treat for dry skin, enriched with **shea butter**, **olive oil**, and **coconut oil**—ingredients that deeply moisturize and nourish. The addition of **rose clay** and **fresh ginger root** provides detoxifying and soothing benefits, making it perfect for replenishing dry skin and leaving it soft, smooth, and radiant.

Oily and Acne-Prone Skin

If you have **oily** or **acne-prone skin**, finding the right balance can sometimes feel tricky. You need a soap that cleanses deeply while keeping excess oil in check, without leaving your skin feeling dry or irritated.

- **Recommended Soap: Lemon Butter**
    - **Why It Works**: Our **Lemon Butter** soap features **fresh lemon**, which has natural astringent properties that help control oil and balance your skin's moisture levels.

Combined with **organic shea butter**, **coconut oil**, and **olive oil**, this soap offers a refreshing deep cleanse while preventing excess oil buildup. It's the perfect solution for clearer, smoother skin, with the added bonus of calming essential oils.

Sensitive Skin

Sensitive skin requires extra care and love. You deserve a soap that's as gentle as it is effective—one that will soothe, calm, and nourish without causing redness or irritation.

- **Recommended Soap: 50:50 Butter**
  - **Why It Works**: With just two natural ingredients—**shea butter** and **coconut oil**—our **50:50 Butter** soap is incredibly gentle and free from harsh additives. It's the ultimate choice for sensitive skin, offering a calming, soothing cleanse that nourishes without irritation, keeping your skin feeling soft and happy.

Combination Skin

If you have **combination skin**, you may notice that some areas are oily (often the T-zone), while others are drier or normal. Finding the right balance is key, and you need a soap that cleanses without over-drying or making certain areas too oily.

- **Recommended Soap: Lemon Butter**
  - **Why It Works**: The **Lemon Butter** soap is perfect for combination skin, as it gently balances oil production while providing hydration where needed. The **lemon** helps control excess oil, while **shea butter**, **coconut oil**, and **olive oil** nourish the drier areas of your skin, leaving it feeling balanced, refreshed, and glowing.

In this book, we'll help you discover the beauty of caring for your skin naturally, with simple, effective solutions tailored to your unique needs. Get ready to fall in love with your skin all over again, with products that are as luxurious as they are pure.

Chapter 1: Understanding Your Skin

Your skin is more than just an outer covering; it's a complex, multifunctional organ that plays a crucial role in maintaining your overall health and well-being. To properly care for your skin, it's essential to understand its structure and how each part functions in harmony to protect and regenerate the body. This knowledge is the foundation for creating an effective skincare routine that nourishes your skin and helps it thrive.

The Structure of Skin: Layers and Functions

The skin is made up of three primary layers, each with a specific function that contributes to the health of your entire body:

1. **Epidermis**:
   The **epidermis** is the outermost layer and your skin's first line of defense. It acts as a protective shield against environmental factors such as bacteria, chemicals, and pollutants. The epidermis is constantly shedding dead skin cells and generating new ones, ensuring your skin remains healthy and resilient over time.

2. **Dermis**:
   Beneath the epidermis lies the **dermis**, which provides strength and flexibility to the skin. This layer is rich in **collagen** and **elastin** fibers, which give skin its elasticity and firmness. The dermis also houses important structures like hair follicles, sweat glands, and blood vessels, which help regulate body temperature and deliver nutrients to the skin.

3. **Hypodermis (Subcutaneous Fat Layer)**:
    The **hypodermis** is the deepest layer of the skin, made up mostly of fat cells. It provides insulation, helps cushion the body from physical impacts, and stores energy. This layer also plays a role in regulating body temperature by acting as a buffer against external temperatures.

Each layer works together to protect, regenerate, and maintain the body's overall homeostasis. Understanding this structure helps you choose the right skincare products that target specific needs, ensuring your skin remains healthy, balanced, and radiant.

The Skin's Natural Barrier: Protecting What's Within

The skin's natural barrier is part of the **epidermis** and is known as the **stratum corneum**. This layer consists of tightly packed cells, called **corneocytes**, surrounded by lipids that act as a shield, locking in moisture while keeping harmful microorganisms and irritants out. When the skin's barrier is functioning well, it prevents water loss, maintains hydration, and protects against environmental aggressors.

However, this barrier can be compromised by external factors such as pollution, harsh skincare products, or even stress. When damaged, it leads to issues like dryness, irritation, and increased sensitivity. That's why using **all-natural products** that work in harmony with the skin's natural processes is essential. These products help protect and strengthen the skin's barrier, ensuring it stays healthy and resilient.

Common Skin Types and Their Needs

Your skin is as unique as you are, and understanding its specific needs is essential for glowing, healthy skin. Let's explore the four basic skin types, what they need, and the best natural ingredients that will have your skin thanking you. Whether you have normal, dry, oily, or combination skin, there's a natural solution waiting to unlock your skin's radiance.

Normal Skin: Well-Balanced and Resilient

What It Is:
Normal skin is the gold standard of skin types—well-balanced, with a smooth texture, good elasticity, and few imperfections. While this skin type doesn't usually experience major issues, maintaining that balance is key to long-lasting beauty.

Do's:

- Use gentle, hydrating cleansers that don't strip the skin of its natural oils.
- Moisturize daily with lightweight, non-comedogenic natural oils like **jojoba oil** or **rosehip oil**, which help maintain moisture without clogging pores.
- Include a natural toner like **witch hazel** to balance pH levels and provide subtle hydration.

Don'ts:

- Avoid harsh cleansers or scrubs that could disrupt your skin's perfect balance.
- Don't skip the sunscreen if you are a person needing protection from the sun. Opt for a mineral-based sunscreen with **zinc oxide** for natural protection.

Best Natural Products for Normal Skin:

- **Aloe vera-based cleansers**: Aloe gently cleanses while providing hydration and soothing properties.
- **Jojoba oil moisturizers**: Jojoba mimics the skin's natural oils, helping maintain that ideal balance.
- **Rose water toners**: Helps refresh, hydrate, and protect the skin's natural moisture barrier.

Dry Skin: Thirsty for Hydration

What It Is:
Dry skin can feel tight, rough, and may be prone to flaking or sensitivity due to insufficient natural oils. This type of skin craves deep, long-lasting hydration and rich emollients that lock in moisture and strengthen the skin barrier.

Do's:

- Look for products rich in **shea butter** and **coconut oil**, which deeply nourish and restore moisture to dry skin.
- Use a **hyaluronic acid serum** before applying moisturizer—it acts as a sponge, drawing water into your skin and keeping it plump and hydrated.

- Incorporate **ceramides** and **omega-3 fatty acids** into your routine to rebuild and protect the skin's moisture barrier.

Don'ts:

- Avoid hot water when washing your face—it strips away natural oils and exacerbates dryness.
- Stay away from alcohol-based toners or astringents that can dry your skin even more.
- Don't over-exfoliate—use gentle exfoliants like **oatmeal scrubs** no more than twice a week.

Best Natural Products for Dry Skin:

- **Shea butter creams**: Rich in fatty acids, shea butter deeply moisturizes, soothes irritation, and provides long-lasting hydration.
- **Coconut oil moisturizers**: Antibacterial and intensely hydrating, coconut oil helps replenish the skin's lipid barrier.
- **Honey-based masks**: Honey is a natural humectant that attracts moisture to the skin, leaving it soft and hydrated.

Oily Skin: Balancing the Shine

What It Is:
Oily skin tends to produce excess sebum, resulting in shine, enlarged pores, and occasional breakouts. But oily skin doesn't mean you should strip away all moisture. The goal is balance—keeping oil in check without over-drying your skin.

Do's:

- Cleanse with **clay-based** or **activated charcoal cleansers** to absorb excess oil and draw out impurities.
- Use lightweight, **water-based moisturizers** or **aloe vera gel** to hydrate without clogging pores.
- Incorporate **tea tree oil** as a spot treatment—its antibacterial properties can help clear up acne and reduce inflammation.

Don'ts:

- Avoid alcohol-based products that can trigger your skin to produce more oil.
- Don't over-cleanse or scrub vigorously, as this will strip the skin of its natural oils and lead to overcompensation (more oil production).
- Stay away from thick, heavy creams or oil-based foundations.

Best Natural Products for Oily Skin:

- **Kaolin clay masks**: Gentle on the skin, kaolin helps absorb excess oil without stripping your skin.
- **Tea tree oil serums**: Known for its antibacterial properties, tea tree oil helps reduce breakouts and keeps skin clear.
- **Witch hazel toners**: A natural astringent, witch hazel tightens pores and reduces oil production.

Combination Skin: Balancing Two Worlds

What It Is:
Combination skin is a mix of dry and oily areas—typically, the T-zone (forehead, nose, chin) is oily, while the cheeks and other areas are dry. This skin type requires a tailored approach that addresses both concerns simultaneously.

Do's:

- Use a **gentle, balancing cleanser** that removes oil from the T-zone while hydrating the drier areas.
- Spot-treat oily areas with **clay masks** and use **hyaluronic acid serums** to hydrate dry zones.
- Opt for **light, gel-based moisturizers** for the oily areas and richer creams for the dry areas.

Don'ts:

- Avoid one-size-fits-all products that could make the oily areas too shiny or the dry areas more parched.
- Don't use heavy creams across your entire face— stick to lighter options for oily areas.
- Avoid over-exfoliating, as it can irritate both dry and oily parts.

Best Natural Products for Combination Skin:

- **Green tea-based cleansers**: Green tea is great for balancing oil production and providing antioxidants.
- **Jojoba oil**: This natural oil mimics your skin's own sebum and works wonders for both oily and dry areas.
- **Rosehip oil**: Lightweight yet deeply nourishing, rosehip oil can hydrate dry areas without clogging the oily parts.

The Path to Glowing, Healthy Skin

Understanding your skin type is the first step in creating a skincare routine that supports your skin's natural processes. With the right combination of natural products and mindful habits, you can achieve balanced, radiant, and healthy skin—no matter your skin type. By embracing nature's finest ingredients and following these do's and don'ts, you'll keep your skin in harmony with its unique needs.

Chapter 2: Factors Contributing to Healthy Skin

Healthy, radiant skin is no accident—it's the result of a balanced lifestyle, nourishing products, and thoughtful care. Everything from the foods you eat to the daily skincare routine you follow has a direct impact on how your skin looks and feels. At **Health Is Luxury**, we know that glowing skin comes from treating it with love, from the inside out. Let's explore the key factors that contribute to vibrant, healthy skin.

Nutrition and Skin Health

The saying "you are what you eat" couldn't be more true when it comes to your skin. Your skin reflects your overall health, and proper nutrition gives it the building blocks it needs to stay strong, smooth, and radiant. What you eat plays a crucial role in your skin's ability to repair itself, regenerate, and fight off damage.

- **Vitamins:**
  Vitamins A, C, D, and E are essential for healthy skin. For example, **Vitamin C** helps your skin produce collagen—the protein responsible for keeping skin firm, smooth, and youthful. Meanwhile, **Vitamin E** protects against environmental stressors, like UV rays, that can cause damage and accelerate aging. Including plenty of colorful fruits and vegetables in your diet is a delicious way to boost your vitamin intake and nourish your skin from within.

- **Healthy Fats**:
  Fats often get a bad rap, but **Omega-3 fatty acids**—found in foods like salmon, flaxseeds, and walnuts—are actually skin's best friend. These healthy fats support the skin's **lipid barrier**, helping to lock in moisture and keep your skin hydrated. They also reduce inflammation, which is key for soothing irritated or sensitive skin.

- **Antioxidants**:
  Antioxidants are your skin's natural defenders. Found in berries, green tea, and leafy greens, these powerful compounds fight off free radicals—unstable molecules that damage cells and speed up aging. By loading up on antioxidant-rich foods, you're giving your skin the protection it needs to stay youthful and radiant.

- **Hydration**:
  Water is the ultimate beauty secret. Drinking plenty of water throughout the day ensures your skin stays hydrated from within, improving elasticity and keeping it smooth and supple. Proper hydration also helps detoxify the body, which means fewer impurities that could otherwise cause breakouts or dullness. Hydrated skin is happy skin!

A balanced diet rich in vitamins, minerals, healthy fats, and hydration is essential for skin that looks and feels its best. Your skin is like a garden—what you feed it determines how it blooms.

The Role of Vitamins and Minerals

Vitamins and minerals are like superheroes for your skin. They play a vital role in everything from collagen production to protecting your skin against damage caused by environmental stressors. Let's take a look at a few key players in the world of skin health:

- **Vitamin A**:
  Vitamin A is known for its role in **skin regeneration** and repair. It helps your skin renew itself, making it a must-have for preventing wrinkles and reducing the appearance of fine lines. Foods rich in Vitamin A include carrots, sweet potatoes, and dark leafy greens.

- **Vitamin C**:
  A true multitasker, **Vitamin C** is one of the most powerful antioxidants. It helps protect your skin from harmful free radicals and boosts collagen production, which keeps your skin firm and plump. Citrus fruits, berries, and broccoli are all great sources of Vitamin C.

- **Vitamin E**:
  Often called the "skin vitamin," **Vitamin E** works to protect your skin from UV damage while helping to maintain its moisture balance. Foods like almonds, avocados, and sunflower seeds are rich in this skin-loving vitamin.

- **Zinc**:
  Zinc is an anti-inflammatory mineral that supports the immune system and plays a key role in skin healing. This makes it particularly helpful for **acne-prone** skin. You can find zinc in pumpkin seeds, quinoa, and lentils.

By incorporating these essential vitamins and minerals into your diet, you're giving your skin everything it needs to stay healthy, strong, and glowing.

Hydration: Inside and Out

When it comes to maintaining healthy skin, **hydration** is key. Hydrated skin looks plumper, feels softer, and has a natural glow that no makeup can replicate. But staying hydrated isn't just about drinking water—it's also about using products that help your skin retain moisture.

- **Internal Hydration**:
  Drinking plenty of water throughout the day is the foundation of hydrated skin. Proper hydration helps keep your skin cells full of moisture, improving their elasticity and overall texture. Plus, it supports your body's natural detoxification processes, helping to flush out toxins that can affect your skin's appearance.

- **External Hydration**:
  Using moisturizers with hydrating ingredients like **hyaluronic acid**, **glycerin**, and **shea butter** helps lock in moisture and prevent water loss from your skin's surface. These ingredients create a barrier that protects your skin from the drying effects of the environment, while also leaving it feeling smooth, soft, and radiant.

When your skin is properly hydrated, it's better equipped to defend itself from external stressors, maintain its elasticity, and reduce the appearance of fine lines and wrinkles. Think of hydration as the foundation for glowing, youthful skin— inside and out.

By paying attention to the foods you eat, staying hydrated, and using the right skincare products, you can create the perfect environment for your skin to flourish. Healthy, glowing skin is within reach, and it all starts with nourishing it from the inside out.

Chapter 3: The Importance of Blood Health in Skincare

Healthy, glowing skin isn't just about what you put on the surface—it's also deeply connected to what's happening inside your body. One of the most important, yet often overlooked, factors in maintaining radiant skin is the health of your blood. Your blood nourishes your skin from within, delivering oxygen and essential nutrients while carrying away toxins. When your blood is healthy and clean, your skin reflects that vitality, radiating a natural glow. Let's explore the powerful link between blood health and skincare, and discover how caring for your blood can lead to clearer, more vibrant skin.

Blood's Role in Nourishing the Skin

Your skin is constantly renewing itself, shedding old cells and generating new ones. This process is powered by the blood, which acts as a delivery system for vital nutrients and oxygen that your skin needs to stay healthy and youthful. The circulatory system ensures that these essential elements reach even the outermost layers of your skin, keeping your complexion smooth, clear, and vibrant.

When your blood is rich in nutrients, your skin flourishes, appearing smooth and radiant. On the other hand, if your blood is overloaded with toxins or lacking in essential nutrients, it can show up on your skin as acne, dullness, or premature aging. By focusing on your blood health, you're not only boosting your overall well-being but giving your skin the nourishment it craves.

What Contributes to Healthy Blood?

Maintaining clean, healthy blood is essential for glowing skin, and it all starts with giving your body the right nutrients while minimizing exposure to toxins. Here are a few key factors that contribute to blood health:

- **Nutrient-Rich Diet**:
  Your diet plays a big role in the health of your blood. Foods that are rich in **vitamins**, **minerals**, and **antioxidants**—such as leafy greens, legumes, and beets —help maintain healthy blood flow. For example, **iron** is crucial for the production of hemoglobin, which carries oxygen to your skin cells, keeping them energized and vibrant.

- **Hydration**:
  Water is essential for maintaining blood fluidity and for detoxifying the body. Staying hydrated ensures that your kidneys can flush out waste products, preventing toxins from building up in your bloodstream and affecting your skin.

- **Detoxification**:
  Your liver and kidneys work hard to filter toxins from your blood, keeping your system clean. Supporting these organs by eating foods that enhance detoxification—like **broccoli**, **kale**, and **garlic**—can help purify your blood and promote clearer, healthier skin.

- **Oxygenation**:
  Regular physical activity improves circulation, ensuring that oxygen and nutrients are efficiently delivered to your skin cells. Even **deep breathing exercises** can increase the oxygen content in your blood, giving your skin an instant boost of vitality.

How Toxins and Poor Diet Affect Blood and Skin Health

When your blood becomes overwhelmed by toxins—
whether from processed foods, environmental pollutants, or
stress—it can lead to inflammation and other skin issues.
Here are some common sources of toxins and their impact
on the skin:

- **Processed Foods**:
  Diets high in processed foods, sugars, and
  unhealthy fats can overload your system with
  toxins, making it harder for your liver and kidneys
  to keep your blood clean. This can result in
  breakouts, dullness, and premature aging.

- **Environmental Pollutants**:
  Exposure to chemicals and pollutants in the air,
  water, and food can seep into your bloodstream,
  affecting not only your overall health but also your
  skin.

- **Stress**:
  Chronic stress can trigger the release of hormones
  like **cortisol**, which affects blood circulation and
  increases inflammation. This can lead to breakouts,
  redness, and dull skin.

When your blood is overloaded with toxins, your skin is
often the first place to show signs of distress. Acne,
dullness, and premature aging are just a few of the skin
issues linked to toxin buildup in the bloodstream.

How Clean Blood Leads to Clear, Radiant Skin

Keeping your blood clean and rich in nutrients is one of the most powerful ways to achieve clear, glowing skin. When your blood is free from toxins and full of oxygen, your skin cells are better nourished, allowing them to function at their best. Clean blood helps your skin:

- **Regenerate and Repair**:
  Well-nourished skin cells renew themselves more efficiently, reducing the appearance of blemishes, dark spots, and wrinkles.

- **Stay Hydrated**:
  Good circulation ensures that moisture reaches your skin's outer layers, keeping it soft, supple, and hydrated.

- **Fight Inflammation**:
  Blood that is free from toxins helps prevent inflammatory skin conditions like **acne**, **eczema**, and **rosacea**.

Practical Tips for Keeping Your Blood Clean

You don't need drastic measures to keep your blood clean —just a few simple lifestyle changes can make a big difference. Here are some practical tips to help you maintain healthy blood and glowing skin:

- **Eat a Clean, Balanced Diet**:
  Focus on whole foods that are rich in antioxidants, vitamins, and minerals. **Leafy greens**, **berries**, and **cruciferous vegetables** support detoxification and help purify the blood.

- **Stay Hydrated**:
  Drinking enough water each day helps flush toxins from your system, improving circulation and ensuring that your skin stays hydrated.

- **Exercise Regularly**:
  Physical activity boosts circulation and oxygenates the blood, helping to deliver essential nutrients to your skin cells. Even moderate exercise can make a big difference.

- **Support Detoxification with Herbal Teas**:
  Herbs like **dandelion, burdock root**, and **milk thistle** are known for their blood-purifying properties. Drinking herbal teas made from these ingredients can support liver function and improve both blood and skin health.

- **Avoid Toxins**:
  Reduce your exposure to toxins by choosing **organic foods**, drinking filtered water, and using all-natural skincare products free from harmful chemicals.

Skin Conditions Linked to Poor Blood Health

Certain skin conditions can worsen or develop when blood health is compromised. Here are a few examples:

- **Acne**:
  A buildup of toxins in the blood can lead to inflammation in the skin, causing clogged pores and acne breakouts.

- **Eczema and Psoriasis**:
  These inflammatory skin conditions are often aggravated by a high level of toxins in the bloodstream.

- **Rosacea**:
  Poor circulation and inflammation in the blood vessels can trigger flare-ups in people with rosacea.

Natural Methods to Cleanse the Blood

There are plenty of natural ways to keep your blood clean and support glowing skin. Here are a few simple methods to try:

- **Green Leafy Vegetables**:
  Rich in **chlorophyll**, vegetables like **spinach**, **kale**, and **collard greens** help detoxify the blood by removing toxins and heavy metals.

- **Lemon Water**:
  Starting your day with a glass of warm water and fresh lemon juice can help flush out toxins, alkalize your blood, and improve digestion.

- **Turmeric**:
  This potent anti-inflammatory spice supports liver function and aids in detoxifying the blood.

- **Burdock Root**:
  Known for its blood-purifying properties, **burdock root** helps clear the bloodstream of toxins and reduce skin inflammation.

The Role of Antioxidants in Blood Health

Antioxidants are crucial for protecting your skin from the harmful effects of **free radicals**, which can damage cells and accelerate aging. When your blood is rich in antioxidants, it helps neutralize these free radicals, reducing their impact on your skin. Foods like **blueberries**, **pomegranates**, and **green tea** are packed with antioxidants that support both blood and skin health.

Conclusion: A Holistic Approach to Skin and Blood Health

The connection between blood health and skin health is undeniable. Keeping your blood clean, oxygenated, and nutrient-rich is key to achieving clear, radiant skin. By nourishing your body with the right foods, staying hydrated, and supporting detoxification through natural remedies, you can promote healthy circulation and glowing skin from within. Remember, beautiful skin starts with a healthy, happy body.

Chapter 4: Maintaining Skin Health Naturally

In today's fast-paced world, your skin faces a constant barrage of environmental stressors—pollutants, chemicals, and toxins that can weaken its natural defenses. While many commercial skincare products promise quick fixes, they often rely on harsh synthetic ingredients that disrupt your skin's delicate balance. At **Health Is Luxury**, we believe the secret to long-term skin health lies in the power of all-natural ingredients that work *with* your skin, not against it.

By embracing natural skincare, you can support your skin's ability to repair, rejuvenate, and defend itself—without the risks of irritation, allergic reactions, or long-term damage that come from synthetic chemicals. Pure, plant-based ingredients nourish your skin from the outside in, while protecting it from harmful substances that can weaken its natural barrier.

The Skin's Natural Barrier and Why It Matters

Your skin's natural barrier is a superhero layer called the **stratum corneum**, the outermost layer that shields your body from the outside world. It's made up of tightly packed skin cells and lipids (fats) that keep moisture in and harmful substances out. When this barrier is healthy, your skin stays hydrated, elastic, and resilient against external irritants.

However, many commercial skincare products—especially those containing synthetic chemicals like **EDTA**(ethylenediaminetetraacetic acid)—can compromise this natural barrier. EDTA is often used to improve lathering and extend the shelf life of soaps and cosmetics, but it comes at a cost to your skin's integrity.

The Dangers of EDTA and Synthetic Chemicals

Despite being widely used, **EDTA** poses several risks to the skin. It weakens the skin's permeability, making it easier for harmful substances to penetrate, especially considering the increasing levels of toxins in public water systems, like heavy metals and chlorine.

When your skin barrier is compromised by EDTA or similar synthetic chemicals, it becomes more vulnerable to environmental toxins. This can lead to:

- **Irritation and Inflammation**: Particularly for sensitive or eczema-prone skin, which relies on a strong barrier to prevent irritation.
- **Disruption of the Skin's Microbiome**: The skin's microbiome is a natural layer of beneficial bacteria that protects against pathogens and helps retain moisture. When this balance is disrupted, skin becomes prone to dryness and infection.
- **Increased Absorption of Toxins**: Weakened skin barriers allow more environmental toxins to enter, leading to long-term damage.

But EDTA isn't the only harmful ingredient. Many commercial soaps, creams, and lotions contain a cocktail of synthetic chemicals that may compromise your skin's health over time.

Other Harmful Toxins Found in Commercial Skincare Products

While EDTA is one concern, there are plenty of other synthetic ingredients lurking in everyday skincare products that may be doing more harm than good. Here are some common toxins found in commercial soaps, lotions, and creams that are worth avoiding:

- **Parabens**:
  Parabens are preservatives used in many skincare products to extend their shelf life. However, they're known to disrupt hormones and have been linked to an increased risk of breast cancer. Parabens can also cause allergic reactions and skin irritation.

- **Sulfates (Sodium Lauryl Sulfate/Sodium Laureth Sulfate)**:
  Commonly found in soaps, shampoos, and cleansers, sulfates are harsh detergents that strip the skin of its natural oils, leading to dryness, irritation, and even eczema flare-ups.

- **Phthalates**:
  Phthalates are used to make fragrances last longer, but they're also endocrine disruptors, meaning they can interfere with your body's hormone balance. Over time, phthalates can cause allergic reactions and skin sensitivities.

- **Artificial Fragrances**:
  Synthetic fragrances are a blend of undisclosed chemicals that can cause allergic reactions, headaches, and skin irritation. Unlike natural essential oils, these artificial scents don't offer any skin benefits and can actually contribute to long-term sensitivity.

- **Triclosan**:
  Used in antibacterial soaps and creams, **triclosan** has been linked to skin irritation and hormone disruption. Its overuse can also lead to the development of antibiotic-resistant bacteria, making it an unnecessary risk for your skin.

By using products with these harmful ingredients, you may unknowingly be weakening your skin's defenses, leaving it vulnerable to damage, inflammation, and aging. That's why switching to natural, plant-based skincare is one of the best things you can do for your skin.

The Benefits of Natural Soaps

Natural soaps are a powerful way to cleanse and nourish your skin without disrupting its protective barrier. At **Health Is Luxury**, our handmade soaps are crafted with pure, organic ingredients like **shea butter**, **coconut oil**, and **olive oil**, which work to strengthen and hydrate your skin.

- **Gentle Cleansing Without Stripping**:
  Unlike synthetic soaps, which can strip your skin of its natural oils, our natural soaps cleanse gently, preserving your skin's lipid barrier. This helps lock in moisture and keeps your skin hydrated and resilient.

- **Rich in Nutrients**:
  Ingredients like **shea butter** and **coconut oil** are packed with essential fatty acids, vitamins, and antioxidants that nourish the skin deeply, promote healing, and reduce inflammation. These nutrients give your skin a healthy glow.

- **Free from Harmful Additives**:
  Our natural soaps contain no preservatives, artificial fragrances, or chemicals like EDTA. They're designed to be gentle, making them suitable for even the most sensitive skin types.

How Toxins in Public Water Impact Your Skin

In addition to the toxins found in commercial skincare products, the public water system is another source of exposure that can harm your skin. Many public water systems, especially in urban areas, contain contaminants such as:

- **Chlorine and Chloramines**:
  These chemicals are added to disinfect water but can dry out and irritate your skin.

- **Heavy Metals**:
  Trace amounts of **lead**, **mercury**, and **arsenic** can be found in public water supplies. When absorbed through compromised skin, these metals contribute to inflammation, premature aging, and skin damage.

- **Pesticides and Chemical Residues**:
  These substances, often found in agricultural runoff, can disrupt your body's endocrine system and damage your skin's cells.

When your skin's natural barrier is weakened by synthetic chemicals, it becomes even more permeable to these toxins, which can accelerate skin damage and contribute to dryness, irritation, and premature aging.

How Natural Ingredients Combat Environmental Toxins

At **Health Is Luxury**, we believe in the power of organic, plant-based ingredients that don't just cleanse the skin but also act as a shield against environmental toxins:

- **Shea Butter**:
  Rich in fatty acids and vitamins A and E, shea butter helps rebuild the skin's lipid barrier and locks in moisture, making your skin more resilient to external pollutants.

- **Coconut Oil**:
  With its natural antimicrobial properties, coconut oil supports the skin's defense system, protecting against harmful bacteria and environmental stressors.

- **Olive Oil**:
  Olive oil is packed with antioxidants that neutralize free radicals, which are abundant in polluted environments. It also hydrates and soothes the skin, making it a powerful ally against dryness and irritation.

Conclusion: The Natural Path to Skin Health

In a world filled with environmental pollutants and harsh chemicals, the best way to protect and care for your skin is by embracing natural skincare solutions. By avoiding harmful ingredients like EDTA, parabens, sulfates, and artificial fragrances, and choosing products made from pure, organic ingredients, you can preserve your skin's natural strength and beauty.

At **Health Is Luxury**, we are committed to crafting the finest natural soaps that nourish and protect your skin, ensuring it stays healthy, radiant, and resilient. By nurturing your skin with nature's best, you're not only cleansing the surface but also supporting its long-term health and vitality—naturally.

Chapter 5: Herbs, Vitamins, and Natural Ingredients for Radiant Skin

When it comes to achieving glowing, healthy skin, nature has given us an abundance of powerful tools. Vitamins, minerals, and herbs provide essential nutrients that support the skin's natural regeneration process, keeping it hydrated, nourished, and protected from the elements. At **Health Is Luxury**, we celebrate the richness of these natural ingredients, knowing they are key to long-term skin health and radiance.

Let's explore some of the most effective natural ingredients and how they can transform your skincare routine.

Vitamins for Healthy, Glowing Skin

Vitamins are nature's gift to your skin, offering everything from repair to protection. Incorporating these essential nutrients into your diet and skincare products can make a world of difference for your complexion.

- **Vitamin A: The Skin Repair Vitamin**
  Benefits: Vitamin A is a skin-rejuvenating powerhouse. It boosts cell turnover, helping prevent clogged pores and promoting smoother, more even skin. It's also a fantastic anti-aging ally, reducing the appearance of fine lines and wrinkles over time.
  Natural Sources: Sweet potatoes, carrots, and spinach are packed with Vitamin A. For topical use, look for natural skincare products containing **retinoids** (a derivative of Vitamin A) for an extra boost in skin repair and renewal.

- **Vitamin C: The Collagen Booster**
  Benefits: Vitamin C is essential for **collagen production**, the protein responsible for keeping your skin firm, elastic, and youthful. It also brightens your complexion, reduces pigmentation, and protects against environmental stressors.
  Natural Sources: Citrus fruits, strawberries, and bell peppers are great dietary sources of Vitamin C. For a more targeted approach, using a **Vitamin C serum** in your skincare routine can help promote a radiant, glowing complexion.

- **Vitamin E: The Antioxidant Protector**
  Benefits: Vitamin E is a powerful **antioxidant** that helps protect your skin from damage caused by UV rays, pollution, and other environmental stressors. It also supports skin healing and keeps your skin hydrated.
  Natural Sources: Incorporate more nuts, seeds, and avocados into your diet to enjoy Vitamin E's benefits. **Vitamin E oil** is also excellent for moisturizing and reducing the appearance of scars.

- **Zinc: The Anti-Inflammatory Mineral**
  Benefits: Zinc is a great ingredient for those with **acne-prone skin** because it helps regulate oil production while supporting the skin's immune response. It also aids in the healing of damaged or inflamed skin.
  Natural Sources: Pumpkin seeds, chickpeas, and lentils are rich in zinc and make great additions to your diet for skin health.

Herbs for Radiant Skin

Herbs are another incredible resource for healthy, vibrant skin. These plant-based wonders offer a range of soothing, healing, and protective properties that can enhance your skincare routine naturally.

- **Aloe Vera:**
  Known for its soothing and healing properties, **aloe vera** is ideal for hydrating and calming irritated skin. Whether you've spent too much time in the sun or your skin needs extra moisture, aloe vera offers gentle, nourishing care.

- **Calendula:**
  Calendula has anti-inflammatory and antibacterial properties, making it an effective remedy for treating minor wounds, soothing eczema, and combating acne. It's a gentle yet powerful herb that supports skin healing and reduces inflammation.

- **Chamomile:**
  Chamomile is a natural anti-inflammatory that helps soothe sensitive or irritated skin. If your skin feels stressed, chamomile's calming properties can provide relief and restore balance.

- **Green Tea:**
  Rich in antioxidants, **green tea** is a fantastic ingredient for fighting free radicals and reducing inflammation. It promotes youthful, radiant skin by neutralizing harmful environmental stressors that can lead to aging.

Natural Oils and Butters for Skin Health

Natural oils and butters are packed with nourishing fatty acids, vitamins, and antioxidants that deeply moisturize and protect your skin. These plant-based ingredients are gentle on your skin and provide long-lasting hydration, making them staples in any natural skincare routine.

- **Coconut Oil**:
  Coconut oil is rich in fatty acids that deeply moisturize your skin, creating a protective barrier that helps retain moisture. It also has **antimicrobial properties**, making it a fantastic option for soothing irritated or acne-prone skin.

- **Shea Butter**:
  Shea butter is loaded with vitamins and fatty acids that nourish your skin and protect its natural barrier. It's incredibly moisturizing, helping to heal dry or damaged skin while restoring softness and elasticity.

- **Rosehip Oil**:
  Full of antioxidants and essential fatty acids, **rosehip oil** helps brighten your complexion and reduce the appearance of scars and wrinkles. It's a luxurious addition to any skincare routine, offering both hydration and anti-aging benefits.

Conclusion: Harnessing Nature's Power for Radiant Skin

At **Health Is Luxury**, we believe that the best skincare comes from nature itself. By incorporating these vitamins, herbs, and natural oils into your daily routine, you can nourish your skin deeply, protect it from environmental damage, and support its natural ability to heal and regenerate.

Whether you're looking to brighten, hydrate, or soothe your skin, nature has the perfect solution. Embrace the power of natural ingredients and discover how they can transform your skin into a radiant, glowing canvas.

Chapter 6: The Role of All-Natural Soaps in Skincare

Your skin deserves the very best, and when it comes to choosing the right soap, not all options are created equal. **All-natural soaps,** like those crafted by **Health Is Luxury,** offer nourishment, protection, and a harmonious relationship with your skin—leaving it soft, radiant, and glowing. Synthetic soaps, on the other hand, are packed with harmful chemicals that disrupt your skin's natural balance, stripping away essential oils and leaving your skin vulnerable. Let's dive into why **natural is better** and how our luxurious soaps can transform your skincare routine.

Why Synthetic Soaps Harm the Skin

Commercial, synthetic soaps may seem convenient, but they come with a hidden cost: the health of your skin. These soaps are often filled with detergents, sulfates, and preservatives designed to create a rich lather, but these ingredients can actually damage your skin.

Here's what synthetic soaps do to your skin:

- **Disrupt the Skin's pH Balance**: Synthetic soaps often have a high pH that can disrupt the natural balance of your skin, leading to dryness, irritation, and even inflammation.

- **Strip Away Natural Oils**: Your skin produces oils to protect itself, but synthetic soaps can strip these oils away, leaving your skin dry, tight, and more susceptible to environmental damage.

- **Introduce Harmful Toxins**: Many synthetic soaps contain harmful chemicals like parabens and sulfates, which can penetrate the skin and cause long-term damage, including premature aging and irritation.

The truth is, what you put on your skin matters just as much as what you put in your body. That's why at **Health Is Luxury**, we believe in harnessing the power of **pure, natural ingredients** to create a soap that not only cleanses but nourishes.

Health Is Luxury: Crafting the World's Best Soap

At **Health Is Luxury**, we are dedicated to crafting the finest soaps in the world, using the purest organic ingredients to deliver unmatched results. Our soaps aren't just about cleansing—they're about caring for your skin in a way that maintains its natural beauty and health.

Here's what makes our soap so special:

- **Free from Harsh Chemicals**: We never use artificial fragrances, dyes, or harmful preservatives. Our soaps are perfect for those with sensitive skin, and free from anything that might irritate or disrupt your skin's natural processes.

- **Rich in Moisturizing Ingredients**: Our soaps are packed with nourishing ingredients like **shea butter**, **coconut oil**, and **olive oil**—all of which help keep your skin soft, hydrated, and protected from environmental stressors.

- **Handcrafted with Care**: Every bar of soap we create is carefully crafted to strike the perfect balance between **cleansing** and **moisturizing**. It's gentle enough for daily use yet powerful enough to keep your skin looking and feeling its best.

How to Make Your Skin Beautiful, Soft, and Radiant

Beautiful, radiant skin doesn't just happen overnight—it's the result of consistent care, natural products, and nourishing routines. Here's how you can elevate your skincare routine to achieve glowing, healthy skin every day.

- **Gentle Exfoliation**:
  Exfoliation is key to a smooth, glowing complexion, but it has to be done the right way. Using **natural exfoliants**like **sugar scrubs** or **oatmeal** once or twice a week helps remove dead skin cells without irritating the skin. The result? Brighter, softer skin that's ready to absorb all the goodness of your moisturizing routine.

- **Hydration with Natural Oils**:
  After cleansing, it's essential to **lock in moisture**. Natural oils like **coconut oil**, **jojoba oil**, or **argan oil** are perfect for this—they're easily absorbed, won't clog pores, and work for all skin types. These oils create a protective layer on your skin, keeping it soft, supple, and glowing.

- **Daily Cleansing with Natural Soap**:
  A good skincare routine starts with cleansing, but not just any soap will do. Using **Health Is Luxury's natural soaps** at the end of the day helps remove impurities, pollutants, and makeup without stripping your skin. Our soaps leave your skin feeling clean, soft, and fully hydrated—ready to renew itself overnight.

Consistency Is Key!!

When it comes to achieving and maintaining beautiful skin, consistency is your best friend. Sticking to a routine of **gentle cleansing**, **hydration**, and **protection** is what truly makes the difference over time. Make caring for your skin a daily ritual—a moment of luxury and self-care that you can enjoy while knowing you're using the best products for your skin's long-term health.

At **Health Is Luxury**, we believe that great skin is a reflection of the love and care you give it. With our all-natural soaps and the right routine, you can unlock your skin's full potential, achieving the beautiful, soft, and radiant complexion you've always wanted.

Chapter 7: External and Environmental Factors Affecting Skin Health

Your skin doesn't just reflect what you put on it or eat—it also tells the story of the world around you. Every day, your skin faces a barrage of environmental factors that can either nourish or damage it. From sun exposure to pollutants in the air, these external elements play a huge role in your skin's health. But with the right knowledge and care, you can shield your skin from harm and enhance its natural glow.

Excessive Sun Exposure and Skin Damage

The sun, while essential for life, can be both a friend and a foe to your skin. **UV rays** are one of the biggest culprits behind premature skin aging and damage. Overexposure can have serious consequences, including:

- **Premature Aging**: Sun damage is a leading cause of **wrinkles**, **fine lines**, and **sunspots**. The more UV rays your skin absorbs over time, the quicker it loses elasticity and firmness, leading to a more aged appearance.

- **Hyperpigmentation**: Exposure to UV rays triggers the production of melanin, which can lead to **dark spots** or uneven patches on the skin. This hyperpigmentation can make your complexion appear uneven and dull.

- **Skin Cancer**: Prolonged exposure to UV rays can increase the risk of skin cancer in some individuals. Protecting your skin from the sun is essential for long-term skin health.

The best defense against sun damage is prevention. Always use a natural, broad-spectrum sunscreen, wear protective clothing, and seek shade when the sun is at its peak.

Pollution and Toxins: Invisible Skin Aggressors

Urban environments may provide a vibrant backdrop for life, but the pollutants and toxins in the air are not so kind to your skin. **Air pollution** is filled with free radicals— unstable molecules that can penetrate the skin and cause **oxidative stress**. This leads to premature aging, inflammation, and a weakened skin barrier. Over time, your skin may appear dull, tired, or even irritated.

To combat pollution, using antioxidant-rich products is key. **Antioxidants** neutralize free radicals, preventing them from causing damage and keeping your skin looking healthy and vibrant.

The Gift of Melanin: A Natural Protector

Melanin is more than just the pigment that gives your skin, hair, and eyes their color—it's a natural defense mechanism. Often referred to as a **divine gift**, melanin plays a crucial role in protecting your skin from environmental damage and oxidative stress.

- **Protection from UV Radiation**: Melanin acts as a natural shield, absorbing and dissipating harmful UV rays before they can damage your skin's DNA. People with higher levels of melanin are less susceptible to skin cancer and sunburn because of this protective barrier.

- **Slower Aging Process**: Melanin helps prevent the breakdown of collagen and elastin, the proteins responsible for your skin's firmness and elasticity. This means that people with melanin-rich skin often experience **fewer wrinkles**and signs of aging compared to those with lower melanin levels.

- **Even Skin Tone**: Melanin works to absorb excess UV exposure and spread it evenly across your skin, preventing damage from penetrating too deeply. This helps maintain an **even complexion** and reduces the risk of sunspots or discoloration.

The Pineal Gland: The Powerhouse of Melanin Production

Your body produces melanin through specialized cells known as **melanocytes**, but its production is influenced by the **pineal gland**—an often-overlooked but incredibly powerful gland. Known as the "seat of the soul," the pineal gland regulates important hormones, including melatonin, which works hand-in-hand with melanin to protect your skin and body from oxidative damage.

Taking care of your pineal gland is essential for healthy melanin production. Factors such as diet, lifestyle, and toxin exposure can either boost or inhibit this vital gland's function, which in turn affects your skin's ability to produce melanin effectively.

Nutritional Support for Melanin Production

Nourishing your body from within is key to supporting melanin production and protecting your skin from environmental damage. Certain vitamins, minerals, and amino acids play a significant role in enhancing melanin's protective properties:

- **Vitamin A**: Promotes **cell turnover** and is vital for melanin production. Foods rich in beta-carotene — such as **carrots, sweet potatoes**, and **spinach** — stimulate melanin production, promoting healthy skin and hair pigmentation.

- **Copper**: A trace mineral that's essential for the enzyme tyrosinase, which is crucial for melanin synthesis. **Dark chocolate, almonds**, and **mushrooms** are rich in copper and can help enhance melanin production.

- **Vitamin C**: Supports melanin production by aiding in **iron absorption** and promoting tyrosinase function. **Citrus fruits, berries**, and **broccoli** are excellent sources of Vitamin C, which also helps protect your skin from oxidative stress.

- **Tyrosine**: An amino acid that serves as a building block for melanin. You can find tyrosine in foods like **almonds, avocados, bananas**, and **poultry**, all of which support melanin production and protect the skin.

- **Iron**: Vital for transporting oxygen to skin cells and supporting melanin production. Leafy green vegetables like **spinach** and **kale**, along with **beans** and **lentils**, are excellent sources of iron.

Vitamins and Supplements for Melanin-Rich Skin

Melanin-rich skin has unique needs, especially when it comes to maintaining optimal health and radiance. Proper nutrition and specific supplements can help support your skin's natural beauty.

- **Vitamin D**: Melanin-rich skin naturally produces less Vitamin D when exposed to sunlight, so supplementing with Vitamin D or consuming **fortified foods** like dairy and fish can help maintain healthy levels.

- **Vitamin E**: As a powerful antioxidant, Vitamin E protects melanin-rich skin from environmental damage while supporting the skin's ability to heal. **Almonds**, **sunflower seeds**, and **wheat germ oil** are great sources of Vitamin E.

- **Zinc**: Zinc is essential for **regulating melanin production** and reducing skin inflammation. **Pumpkin seeds**, **chickpeas**, and **whole grains** are excellent dietary sources of zinc.

- **Melatonin Supplements**: Since melatonin is closely linked to melanin production, taking melatonin supplements can help regulate sleep patterns and enhance the body's defense mechanisms. It also contributes to maintaining healthy, youthful skin.

Toxic Skincare Ingredients That May Damage Melanin Production

Toxins in commercial skincare products can disrupt melanin production and damage your skin's natural defenses. Here are some of the most harmful ingredients to avoid:

- **Hydroquinone**: A skin-lightening agent used to treat hyperpigmentation but can lead to the loss of natural melanin over time, resulting in **patchy, uneven skin tone**.

- **Sulfates**: Found in soaps and shampoos, sulfates strip the skin of natural oils and disrupt melanin production, leaving the skin vulnerable to environmental damage.

- **Parabens**: These preservatives can interfere with hormone regulation and melanin synthesis. They can also increase the risk of **skin irritation** and allergic reactions.

- **Mercury**: Found in some unregulated skin-lightening products, mercury is highly toxic and can severely damage melanin production, leading to rashes, discoloration, and scarring.

Protecting and Nourishing Melanin-Rich Skin Naturally

To support and protect your melanin production, choose natural skincare products that work with your skin, not against it. At **Health Is Luxury**, we're committed to using organic, plant-based ingredients that nourish and strengthen your skin.

- **Natural Soaps**: Our soaps are free from harmful chemicals that can interfere with melanin production. Ingredients like **shea butter** and **coconut oil** gently cleanse and hydrate melanin-rich skin.

- **Antioxidant-Rich Formulas**: Our products contain high levels of antioxidants like **Vitamin C** and **Vitamin E**, which protect melanin from oxidative stress and environmental toxins, ensuring your skin stays healthy and vibrant.

The Power of Melanin

Melanin is more than just a pigment—it's a powerful shield, gifted by nature to protect your skin from environmental damage, premature aging, and UV exposure. By nourishing your body with the right nutrients, supporting your pineal gland, and using skincare products free from harmful chemicals, you can enhance your melanin production and keep your skin glowing, even, and resilient.

Melanin is a gift to be celebrated. Through mindful lifestyle choices and natural skincare, you can ensure your melanin-rich skin stays healthy, radiant, and full of life.

Chapter 8: Internal Factors: Gut Health and Skin Health

Your skin is a reflection of what's happening inside your body, and nowhere is this more evident than in the relationship between your **gut** and your skin. Often called the "second brain," the gut plays a central role in everything from **immune function** and **metabolism** to **detoxification**. When your gut is in balance and thriving, the results shine through—literally! Healthy, radiant skin starts from within, with a happy, well-nourished gut. But when your gut is out of sync, skin issues such as acne, inflammation, and even premature aging can arise.

The Gut-Skin Axis: How They Communicate

The connection between your **gut** and **skin**—known as the **gut-skin axis**—is a powerful one. Your gut is home to trillions of microorganisms, known collectively as the **gut microbiome**, which are responsible for everything from digesting food to regulating your immune system. This community of microbes has a profound influence on your skin through several key pathways:

- **Immune Regulation**: A healthy gut microbiome helps to balance your immune system, reducing inflammation and helping to prevent skin conditions such as **acne**, **rosacea**, and **eczema**.

- **Detoxification**: The gut plays a critical role in filtering out toxins from the food you eat. If your gut is imbalanced, these toxins can accumulate, causing **inflammation**, **clogged pores**, and other skin issues.

- **Hormonal Balance**: The gut is involved in regulating hormones like **insulin** and **androgens**, both of which are linked to **acne** and **oily skin**. An unhealthy gut can lead to hormonal imbalances that wreak havoc on your complexion.

By nurturing your gut, you not only support better digestion and overall wellness but also promote **clearer, healthier skin**.

Foods That Promote Glowing Skin

What you eat has a direct impact on your gut health—and in turn, on your skin. Certain foods and nutrients actively support the gut microbiome, leading to clearer, more hydrated, and youthful-looking skin.

- **Probiotic-Rich Foods**:
  Probiotics are live bacteria that help balance your gut microbiome. When your gut is populated with healthy bacteria, inflammation is reduced, and your immune system gets a boost—both of which reflect positively on your skin.
  Sources: Yogurt (with live cultures), **sauerkraut, kimchi, kefir, miso**, and **kombucha**. Regular consumption of these foods helps strengthen the gut-skin connection, keeping skin clear and hydrated.

- **Prebiotics**:
  Prebiotics are non-digestible fibers that act as food for probiotics, helping beneficial bacteria thrive. A diet rich in prebiotics promotes a balanced gut microbiome and clearer skin.
  Sources: Garlic, onions, leeks, asparagus, bananas, and **oats** are excellent sources of prebiotic fibers that nourish gut bacteria and promote clearer, healthier skin.

- **Fiber**:
  A fiber-rich diet is essential for healthy digestion and detoxification. When toxins build up due to poor digestion, they can lead to skin issues like **breakouts, dullness**, and **inflammation.**
  Sources: Whole grains, legumes, fruits, and **vegetables** provide ample fiber to support digestion, encourage regular bowel movements, and help keep skin clear.

- **Omega-3 Fatty Acids**:
  Healthy fats, particularly **omega-3s**, help maintain the skin's lipid barrier, keeping it hydrated, plump, and resilient. Omega-3s also have anti-inflammatory properties, reducing redness, irritation, and acne.
  Sources: Fatty fish (like **salmon, sardines**, and **mackerel**), **chia seeds, flaxseeds, walnuts**, and **hemp seeds** are rich in omega-3s that promote glowing skin and protect it from environmental stressors.

- **Antioxidant-Rich Foods**:
  Antioxidants neutralize free radicals, which can damage skin cells and accelerate aging. A diet rich in antioxidants supports the gut's ability to detoxify harmful compounds and maintain a balanced, glowing complexion.
  Sources: Berries (like **blueberries, strawberries,** and **raspberries**), **leafy greens, green tea**, and **dark chocolate**are loaded with antioxidants that keep skin youthful and vibrant.

Detoxification for Clear Skin

A well-functioning gut plays a vital role in the body's natural **detoxification** processes. When your digestive system is working smoothly, it helps remove waste and toxins, preventing them from being reabsorbed into your bloodstream. But when your gut struggles to eliminate these toxins, they often show up on your skin as **acne**, **dullness**, or **eczema**.

Here's how to support your body's detoxification processes for clearer skin:

- **Hydration**:
  Drinking water is one of the simplest and most effective ways to support detoxification. Water helps flush toxins from your body, keeps digestion running smoothly, and hydrates your skin from within.
  Tip: Aim for at least **8 glasses of water** a day, and consider adding herbal teas like **peppermint**, **ginger**, or **dandelion tea**, which support digestion and detoxification.

- **Herbal Teas**:
  Certain herbs are known for their detoxifying properties and can cleanse the liver, kidneys, and gut. These organs filter out toxins that could otherwise lead to skin inflammation or breakouts.

    - **Dandelion Tea**: A natural diuretic, dandelion tea supports **liver function** and detoxification, promoting clearer skin.
    - **Burdock Root Tea**: Burdock root is known for its **blood-purifying** properties, helping to eliminate toxins and reducing skin conditions like acne and eczema.

- **Fiber-Rich Foods**:
  Fiber is essential for healthy digestion because it promotes regular bowel movements and prevents the buildup of toxins in the gut. A well-functioning digestive system is key to maintaining clear, radiant skin.
  Tip: Incorporate more **whole grains, beans, lentils**, and **vegetables** into your diet to support detoxification.

- **Sweating**:
  Sweating is another way the body eliminates toxins. Regular physical activity, or spending time in a sauna, can help clear your skin by pushing out impurities. Exercise also boosts blood circulation, delivering oxygen and nutrients to your skin cells for a glowing complexion.

The Importance of Gut-Brain-Skin Communication

There's a growing body of research highlighting the interconnectedness of the **gut, brain**, and **skin**. When you experience emotional stress, it directly impacts your gut health, which in turn can lead to **skin issues** like acne, eczema, or rosacea.

- **Mindful Eating**:
  Stressful eating habits can disrupt digestion and nutrient absorption. Eating mindfully—when you're calm and focused—supports both gut health and emotional well-being.

- **Probiotics for Stress Relief**:
  Taking **probiotic supplements** that support gut health may also help reduce stress-related skin problems by improving the **gut-brain-skin** connection. A healthy gut leads to a calmer mind and clearer skin.

Conclusion: A Healthy Gut for Glowing Skin

The connection between your gut and your skin is undeniable. By nourishing your gut with the right foods, supporting digestion and detoxification, and managing stress, you can achieve clearer, more radiant skin. A balanced, healthy gut microbiome is key to a complexion free from inflammation, breakouts, and premature aging. Invest in your gut health, and your skin will thank you.

Chapter 9: Blood Cleansing for Optimal Skin Health

Your skin's health is deeply connected to the health of your blood. Just as your skin relies on external care and nourishment, it also needs a steady supply of **clean, oxygen-rich blood** to look its best. Your blood delivers essential nutrients to skin cells, helps eliminate toxins, and supports the regeneration of new, healthy tissue. When your circulatory system is functioning well, your skin reflects that vitality with a vibrant, glowing appearance. But when toxins build up in the bloodstream, the effects can be seen in **breakouts, dullness,** and **inflammation.**

In this chapter, we explore natural ways to **purify the blood** and enhance skin health using **herbs, chlorophyll-rich foods, intermittent fasting,** and **antioxidants.**

The Importance of Blood Cleansing for Skin Health

The condition of your blood directly affects your skin. Blood transports **oxygen, nutrients,** and **hormones** to your skin cells while removing waste and toxins. When your blood is clean and free of harmful substances, your skin reflects that with a glowing, even complexion. However, when toxins accumulate in the bloodstream, it can lead to a range of skin issues, such as:

- **Inflammation**: Toxins in the blood can cause systemic inflammation, leading to **redness** and **irritation** in the skin.
- **Breakouts**: Impurities in the bloodstream can clog pores, contributing to **acne** and **blemishes.**

- **Dullness**: Without proper nutrients and oxygen, skin can appear **lifeless** and **dull**.

By regularly cleansing your blood, you can:

- **Reduce inflammation**, promoting clearer, calmer skin.
- **Support skin regeneration**, speeding up the healing of damaged skin cells.
- **Promote clear, radiant skin**, free from the toxins that can cause blemishes and dullness.

Chlorophyll-Rich Foods for Blood Purification

Chlorophyll, the green pigment found in plants, is a powerhouse when it comes to purifying the blood. It helps **detoxify**the body, supports **oxygen delivery** to skin cells, and promotes healthy liver function, which is crucial for filtering toxins from the bloodstream. Including chlorophyll-rich foods in your diet can enhance both **blood** and **skin health**.

- **Chlorella**:
  A type of freshwater algae, chlorella is packed with chlorophyll, **vitamins**, **minerals**, and **amino acids**. It helps bind to heavy metals and other toxins, removing them from the bloodstream. Additionally, chlorella's high antioxidant content helps neutralize free radicals, reducing oxidative stress on the skin. **How to Use**: Add chlorella powder to smoothies or juices, or take it in tablet form as a supplement.

- **Spirulina**:
  Another type of algae, spirulina is known as a **superfood** due to its high concentration of **protein**, **vitamins**, **minerals**, and chlorophyll. It helps cleanse the blood by binding to toxins and

enhancing detoxification processes, while also supporting immune health and promoting **glowing skin**.

How to Use: Spirulina can be added to green drinks or smoothies or taken as a supplement in powder or tablet form.

- **Wheatgrass**:
  Rich in chlorophyll and essential nutrients, wheatgrass supports **liver detoxification** and blood purification. Its alkaline properties help reduce **acidity** in the body, which can lead to **skin inflammation**. By increasing oxygen levels in the blood, wheatgrass promotes healthy, radiant skin.
  How to Use: Drink wheatgrass juice or add wheatgrass powder to smoothies for a detoxifying boost.

- **Dark Leafy Greens**:
  Vegetables like **spinach**, **kale**, and **collard greens** are rich in chlorophyll and provide essential **vitamins** and **minerals** for healthy blood and skin. These greens help cleanse the blood by promoting the elimination of toxins through the **liver** and **kidneys**.
  How to Use: Incorporate dark leafy greens into your salads, smoothies, or juices regularly to support blood purification.

Green Drinks for Skin Health

Green drinks are an easy and delicious way to flood your body with chlorophyll, **vitamins**, and **antioxidants** that support both **blood** and **skin health**. A daily green drink made with **chlorella**, **spirulina**, and **dark leafy greens** can help:

- **Detoxify the blood** by removing heavy metals and other toxins.
- **Improve circulation**, ensuring that nutrients and oxygen are delivered to your skin cells.
- **Alkalize the body**, reducing inflammation that can lead to skin issues like **acne** or **eczema**.

Intermittent Fasting for Blood Cleansing and Skin Health

Intermittent fasting is a dietary practice that alternates between periods of eating and fasting. During the fasting window, your body shifts its focus from digestion to **repair** and **detoxification**, giving your liver and kidneys the chance to **filter toxins** from the blood more efficiently. This process not only enhances **blood purification** but also improves **skin clarity**and reduces **inflammation**.

Benefits of Intermittent Fasting for Skin:

- **Enhanced Detoxification**: During fasting, the body accelerates its detoxification processes, clearing out toxins that may be affecting your skin.
- **Reduced Inflammation**: Fasting can reduce systemic inflammation, which is often a root cause of acne, rosacea, and other inflammatory skin conditions.

- **Improved Insulin Sensitivity**: Balanced blood sugar levels are essential for preventing **acne** and excessive **oil production**. Fasting helps balance hormone levels, reducing breakouts.
- **Cellular Repair**: Fasting triggers **autophagy**, a process in which the body breaks down and removes damaged cells, allowing for the regeneration of healthier skin cells.

How to Practice Intermittent Fasting:

- **16:8 Method**: Fast for 16 hours, and eat all your meals within an 8-hour window. This is one of the most popular and manageable fasting schedules.
- **24-Hour Fast**: Once or twice a week, fast for a full 24 hours to allow your body to detoxify and repair fully.

As with any dietary change, it's important to listen to your body and consult with a healthcare professional before starting intermittent fasting.

Antioxidants for Healthy Blood and Skin

Antioxidants are your body's defense against **free radicals**, the unstable molecules that cause oxidative damage to cells. By consuming antioxidant-rich foods, you help keep your blood clean and your skin **clear** and **radiant**.

- **Vitamin C:**
  A potent antioxidant that supports the immune system, helps produce collagen, and protects the skin from **UV damage**.
  Sources: Citrus fruits, strawberries, bell peppers, and broccoli.

- **Green Tea Extract**:
  Loaded with antioxidants, particularly
  epigallocatechin gallate (EGCG), green tea helps
  fight oxidative stress and promotes detoxification.
  How to Use: Drink 2-3 cups of green tea daily or
  take it as a supplement.

- **Quercetin**:
  A flavonoid with anti-inflammatory and antioxidant
  properties, quercetin reduces oxidative damage in
  the blood, improving circulation and promoting
  clear, radiant skin.
  Sources: Apples, onions, berries, and **grapes**.

- **Resveratrol**:
  Found in red grapes, berries, and dark chocolate,
  resveratrol is a powerful antioxidant that reduces
  inflammation and protects the skin from free radical
  damage.
  How to Use: Incorporate resveratrol-rich foods into
  your diet or take a supplement to support both skin
  and blood health.

Additional Natural Practices to Cleanse the Blood

- **Hydration**:
  Drinking plenty of water is essential for blood
  cleansing. Water helps flush toxins from the body,
  keeps the kidneys functioning properly, and ensures
  that your blood stays fluid and clean.

- **Sweating**:
  Engaging in regular physical activity or using a
  sauna helps detoxify the body through sweat. This
  process helps remove toxins that may accumulate in
  the blood, promoting clearer skin.

- **Liver-Supporting Foods**:
  The liver is the body's primary detox organ, and supporting its function is key to keeping your blood clean. Foods like **garlic**, **beets**, and **turmeric** help cleanse the liver and improve its ability to filter toxins from the blood.

Conclusion: The Path to Clean Blood and Healthy Skin

Clean, healthy blood is the foundation of clear, glowing skin. By incorporating **chlorophyll-rich foods**, practicing **intermittent fasting**, and consuming a diet rich in **antioxidants**, you can support your body's natural detoxification processes, ensuring that your blood stays clean and your skin remains radiant. Simple practices like **staying hydrated**, **exercising regularly**, and nourishing your liver with the right foods will help you maintain optimal **blood** and **skin health** for years to come.

Chapter 10: Anti-Aging Through Natural Skincare

Aging is a natural part of life, but it doesn't have to rob your skin of its beauty and vibrancy. By using the right natural ingredients and embracing holistic practices, you can maintain radiant, firm, and youthful skin for longer. In this chapter, we'll explore the power of **antioxidants**, the benefits of **natural ingredients**, and the transformative effects of **meditation** on both the mind and skin.

Natural Antioxidants for Youthful Skin

Antioxidants are essential in the fight against aging. These powerful compounds combat **free radicals**, unstable molecules that accelerate the breakdown of collagen and elastin, leading to wrinkles and sagging. Incorporating antioxidant-rich foods and skincare products into your routine is one of the best ways to defend against environmental stressors and keep your skin looking youthful.

- **Vitamin C**:
  Why It Works: Vitamin C is one of the most potent antioxidants for the skin. It protects against **UV damage**, boosts **collagen production**, and improves **skin texture**. Regular use of Vitamin C helps reduce **dark spots** and **fine lines**, brightening the complexion.
  Sources: Citrus fruits, strawberries, and bell peppers. Topical Vitamin C serums are highly effective for targeting fine lines and sun damage.

- **Vitamin E**:
  Why It Works: Vitamin E is a fat-soluble antioxidant that protects skin cells from oxidative stress while supporting **hydration** and **healing**. It's particularly effective at reducing **scars** and **wrinkles** due to its ability to repair damaged skin.
  Sources: Almonds, sunflower seeds, avocados, and topical Vitamin E oils.

- **Green Tea Extract**:
  Why It Works: Green tea is rich in **polyphenols**, which help fight inflammation and neutralize free radicals. It's proven to reduce visible signs of aging like **wrinkles** and **age spots**, while protecting the skin from UV damage.
  Sources: Drinking green tea or using products with green tea extract provides excellent antioxidant protection.

- **Resveratrol**:
  Why It Works: Found in the skin of grapes, resveratrol smooths **fine lines**, boosts **elasticity**, and protects against environmental damage. It helps preserve collagen and elastin, both essential for keeping skin firm.
  Sources: Red grapes, berries, red wine, and resveratrol supplements or skincare products.

Reversing Damage Naturally

While prevention is essential, it's never too late to reverse some of the visible effects of aging. Using the right **natural ingredients** can help stimulate collagen production, promote **cell turnover**, and deeply nourish the skin, restoring its youthful appearance.

- **Retinol (Vitamin A):**
  Why It Works: Retinol is a well-known anti-aging ingredient that boosts **collagen production**, improves skin texture, and accelerates **cell turnover**. Natural alternatives like **bakuchiol** provide similar benefits without irritation.
  How to Use: Incorporate a natural retinol or bakuchiol serum into your nighttime routine for skin regeneration.

- **Rosehip Oil:**
  Why It Works: Rosehip oil is rich in vitamins A and C, essential fatty acids, and antioxidants. It promotes **collagen production**, fades **dark spots**, smooths **fine lines**, and deeply hydrates.
  How to Use: Apply rosehip oil daily to improve skin elasticity and reduce signs of aging.

- **Shea Butter:**
  Why It Works: Packed with essential fatty acids and vitamins, shea butter restores the skin's moisture barrier, improves softness, and protects against environmental stressors. Its rich, nourishing texture keeps skin plump and hydrated.
  How to Use: Use a moisturizer or body butter with shea butter to lock in hydration and protect your skin.

Building a Routine for Youthful Skin

Creating a consistent, holistic skincare routine is key to keeping your skin looking youthful and vibrant. Incorporate antioxidant-rich ingredients, hydration, and sun protection to prevent premature aging and keep your skin firm and glowing.

- **Daily Cleansing**:
  Use a gentle, natural soap to remove impurities, excess oil, and pollutants. **Health Is Luxury** soaps cleanse without stripping the skin of its natural oils, leaving it hydrated and protected.

- **Moisturizing**:
  Hydration is key to maintaining elasticity and preventing fine lines. Use moisturizers rich in natural oils like **shea butter**, **jojoba oil**, and **argan oil** to nourish the skin and maintain its barrier function.

- **Using Antioxidants**:
  Include antioxidant-rich products like **Vitamin C serums** and **green tea extracts** to protect your skin from free radicals. These antioxidants help prevent wrinkles and sunspots caused by environmental stress.

- **Sun Protection**:
  Protect your skin daily from UV rays with a broad-spectrum sunscreen containing **natural ingredients** like zinc oxide. Sun exposure is a leading cause of premature aging and the breakdown of collagen.

The Power of Meditation for Youthful Skin

Skincare isn't just about what you put on your skin—it's also about how you care for your mind. **Meditation** is a powerful tool for reducing **stress**, which plays a significant role in premature aging. Chronic stress triggers inflammation, breaks down collagen, and reduces circulation to the skin, leading to dullness, fine lines, and wrinkles.

How Stress Affects Skin:

- **Inflammation**: High cortisol levels (the stress hormone) lead to inflammation, causing **acne**, **eczema**, and **rosacea**.
- **Collagen Breakdown**: Cortisol accelerates the breakdown of collagen, leading to **sagging skin**, fine lines, and wrinkles.
- **Reduced Circulation**: Stress reduces blood circulation, depriving the skin of oxygen and nutrients needed for regeneration.

Meditation for Anti-Aging:

Meditation helps calm the mind, reduce stress, and improve overall well-being. This translates into physical benefits for your skin, including improved circulation, reduced inflammation, and better nutrient absorption.

- **Mindful Breathing**: Spend 10-15 minutes a day practicing deep breathing. This reduces cortisol levels and improves blood flow to the skin, giving it a healthy, glowing appearance.

- **Guided Meditation**: Consider adding guided meditation to your daily routine to reduce stress and promote relaxation. There are many apps and resources available to help you start.

- **Gratitude Practice**: Fostering positive emotions through gratitude can help reduce stress, further improving your skin's natural radiance.

Conclusion: A Holistic Approach to Anti-Aging

Achieving youthful skin isn't about one magic product —it's about taking a **holistic approach** that combines natural ingredients with mindful living. By incorporating **antioxidants, collagen-boosting ingredients**, and **meditation** into your routine, you can slow down visible signs of aging and protect your skin from environmental stressors. Take care of your skin, mind, and body, and you'll radiate beauty from the inside out.

Chapter 11: The Holistic Approach to Skincare

At Health Is Luxury, we know that radiant skin is more than just surface-level care. True skin health reflects a balance of **nourishing skincare**, **good nutrition**, **mindful living**, and **emotional well-being**. By embracing a **holistic approach** to skincare, you can transform not only your complexion but your overall health and vitality.

The Mind-Body-Skin Connection

Your skin is a mirror of your internal world. Emotional states like stress, anxiety, and even negative emotions can leave visible marks on your skin, such as **breakouts**, **rashes**, and **premature aging**. The **mind-skin connection** is scientifically proven—your emotions influence the hormones and chemicals your body produces, directly impacting the health of your skin.

How Stress Impacts the Skin:

- **Breakouts and Acne**: When you're stressed, your body produces more **cortisol**, the stress hormone. Elevated cortisol levels stimulate oil production, leading to **clogged pores** and **acne**.
- **Inflammation**: Stress triggers inflammation in the body, worsening conditions like **rosacea**, **eczema**, and **psoriasis**. Chronic stress weakens the skin's natural barrier, making it more vulnerable to damage.
- **Aging**: Cortisol breaks down **collagen**, the protein responsible for keeping skin firm and smooth. High stress levels can accelerate **wrinkles**, **fine lines**, and dullness.

How to Manage Stress for Healthy Skin:

- **Meditation**: Daily meditation calms the mind and body, reducing stress hormones and improving overall skin health. By focusing on **deep breathing** and **mindfulness**, you can lower cortisol levels and support your skin's natural repair process.
- **Breathing Exercises**: Simple, mindful breathing stimulates blood flow to the skin, delivering oxygen and nutrients for a more radiant complexion.
- **Journaling**: Writing down your thoughts and emotions can be a powerful way to release stress. Easing emotional tension promotes a sense of clarity and calm, reflected in a healthier, more balanced complexion.

The Power of Sleep: Beauty Rest for Glowing Skin

Beauty sleep isn't just a saying—it's a necessity! During sleep, your body enters a state of deep **repair** and **regeneration**, where skin cells are renewed, and damage is repaired.

What Happens to Your Skin While You Sleep:

- **Cell Turnover**: Skin cells regenerate faster while you sleep, replacing old, damaged cells with new ones, which promotes a fresher, more vibrant complexion.
- **Collagen Production**: Sleep is when collagen production peaks. Collagen is essential for keeping skin **firm**, **elastic**, and youthful.
- **Hydration Balance**: During sleep, your body balances its hydration levels. Without proper sleep, your skin may become dehydrated, leading to **dark circles**, **puffiness**, and **dryness**.

Tips for Optimizing Your Sleep for Better Skin:

- **Set a Regular Sleep Schedule**: Going to bed and waking up at the same time every day helps your body get the restorative sleep it needs for cell repair and regeneration.
- **Create a Relaxing Sleep Environment**: Dim the lights, lower the room temperature, and eliminate distractions for a restful night's sleep. Consider using **lavender essential oil** to enhance relaxation.
- **Nighttime Skincare Routine**: Before bed, cleanse your skin thoroughly and apply nourishing oils like **rosehip** or **shea butter**. Your skin absorbs nutrients better at night, so hydrating products boost overnight skin repair.

Holistic Skincare: The Health Is Luxury Approach

At Health Is Luxury, we believe that **natural, clean ingredients** paired with mindful practices form the cornerstone of true skincare. Our holistic philosophy is simple: the fewer chemicals you put on your skin, the healthier it will be.

Why Go Natural?:

- **No Harsh Chemicals**: Commercial skincare products often contain synthetic chemicals that strip your skin of its natural oils, irritate sensitive skin, and disrupt its barrier function. Health Is Luxury's natural soaps, made with organic ingredients like **shea butter** and **coconut oil**, cleanse without harm.
- **Nourishing Ingredients**: Natural skincare is packed with powerful plant-based ingredients that work in harmony with your skin's natural processes. For example, **rosehip oil** is rich in vitamins A and C, promoting **collagen production** and reducing fine lines.

- **Eco-Friendly**: Our natural products are better for the environment. Health Is Luxury prioritizes sustainability, using eco-conscious ingredients and packaging that help reduce your carbon footprint.

Creating a Holistic Skincare Routine:

1. **Cleanse**: Start with a gentle, natural soap like our **50:50 Butter**. Avoid cleansers with sulfates and parabens that can strip the skin of its oils.
2. **Exfoliate**: Exfoliate once or twice a week using natural exfoliants like **sugar scrubs** or **oatmeal** to remove dead skin cells and promote cell turnover.
3. **Moisturize**: Use plant-based oils like **jojoba oil**, **shea butter**, or **argan oil** to keep your skin hydrated and protected.
4. **Protect**: Apply a natural sunscreen with **zinc oxide** to protect your skin from harmful UV rays. Sun exposure is one of the leading causes of **premature aging**.

Mindfulness and Skincare: Elevating Your Beauty Rituals

Incorporating **mindfulness** into your skincare routine transforms it from a basic task into a soothing ritual that nurtures your **mind**, **body**, and **spirit**. When you practice mindfulness during your beauty routine, you foster a sense of peace and self-care that boosts not only your skin's health but also your overall well-being.

Mindful Skincare Tips:

- **Be Present**: When you cleanse or moisturize your skin, be fully aware of the sensations and textures. Let go of distractions and focus on the experience. Being present in the moment reduces stress, which positively impacts your skin's health.

- **Affirmations**: As you apply skincare products, repeat positive affirmations like, "My skin is healthy and glowing," or "I am nourishing my body with love." Positive affirmations boost emotional well-being and promote a more loving relationship with your skin.
- **Gratitude Practice**: As you finish your skincare routine, take a moment to express gratitude for your body and skin. Gratitude fosters a deeper connection with yourself, promoting a sense of peace that will radiate through your complexion.

Conclusion: The Path to Long-Term Radiant Skin

At Health Is Luxury, we believe that beautiful skin is a reflection of your inner health and well-being. By embracing a **holistic skincare approach**—one that combines **natural, high-quality ingredients** with **mindful living, stress management**, and **self-care**—you create the foundation for long-term, glowing skin. Simplicity, sustainability, and self-care are the cornerstones of our philosophy, and by incorporating these practices into your daily routine, you're not just enhancing your skin—you're cultivating a **deeper connection** with your body and mind.

www.ingramcontent.com/pod-product-compliance
Lightning Source LLC
Chambersburg PA
CBHW051701090426
42736CB00013B/2493